THE OMAD DIET

BOOK

AN ESSENTIAL GUIDE TO HOW TO BURN FAT,
LOSE WEIGHT, INCREASE YOUR MENTAL
CLARITY AND STAY IN SHAPE
WITH 14 EASY, TASTY, HEALTHY AND
NUTRITIOUS RECIPES FOR ONE MEAL A DAY
PLUS SNACKS

KRISTIN AGING

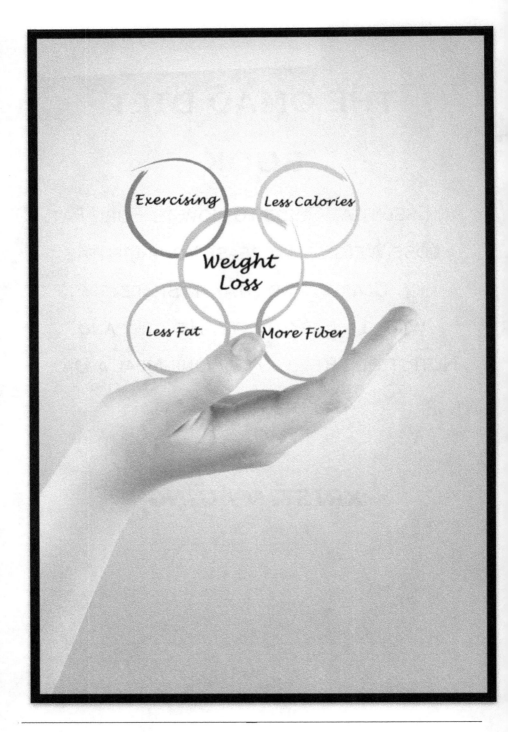

Table Contest

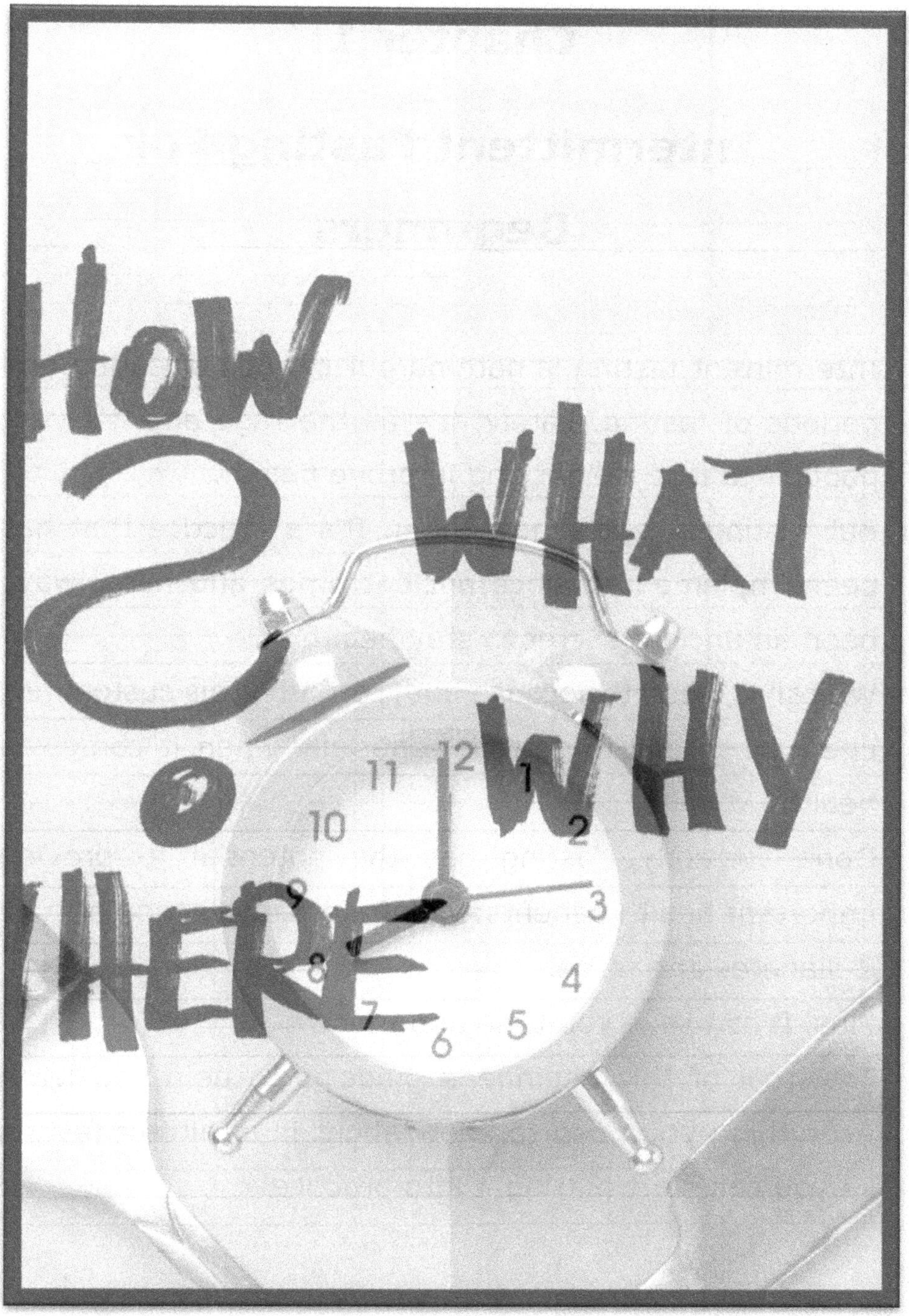
HOW
WHAT
WHY
HERE

Chapter 1:

Intermittent Fasting For Beginners

Intermittent fasting is nothing but periods of eating and periods of fasting. Lately, it's all the rage and it's very popular to lose weight and improve health.

But fasting is not a new thing. It's a practice that has been implemented since ancient times and has always been an ancient secret to stay healthy.

We call it "secret" because until recently, this custom has been practically forgotten, especially when it comes to health.

Done correctly, fasting has the potential to provide important health benefits: weight loss, correction of type 2 diabetes and more.

Plus, it can save you time and money.

The goal of this beginner's guide is to help you learn everything you need to know about intermittent fasting so you can start putting it into practice.

Although intermittent fasting has been shown to offer many benefits, it's still a topic that presents different ideas about its implementation and benefits. Of course, it is always advisable to consult your doctor for any changes in your lifestyle and diet.

I hope that whoever reads this guide, which gives you the basics of what intermittent fasting is, will help you enjoy the health benefits and give you the right information on how to approach this method/diet.
Of course, some people are underweight or have eating disorders such as anorexia or pregnant or nursing women or people under 18 years of age who should not consider it.

Chapter 2:

WHAT IS INTERMITTENT FASTING?

Generally, those who choose to do intermittent fasting are people who are not underweight and therefore have enough stored fat to live with it.

You decide not to eat and you decide the length of the interval to apply, which can be a few hours to days or - with a doctor's supervision - up to a week or more. You can start a fast at any time and you can also stop when you want to. A fast can be started or ended for any reason or no reason at all.

You can decide to fast between dinner and breakfast the next day, an interval of about 12-14 hours. In this sense, fasting can be considered part of daily life.

Intermittent fasting, then, is nothing strange or peculiar, but part of daily life. It is perhaps the oldest and most effective nutritional intervention imaginable.

How Lose weight through intermittent fasting

Basically, fasting allows the body to use stored energy; By eating, more energy is ingested than we can use immediately. Some of this energy must be stored for use later.

It's important to know that this is normal and that humans have evolved to be able to fast for short periods - hours or days - without experiencing harmful effects on our health.

Body fat is just stored food energy. If you don't eat, your body will simply "eat" its fat for energy.

Insulin is the main hormone involved in storing food energy.

Insulin increases when we eat, helping us store excess energy in two different ways. Carbohydrates are broken down into glucose (sugar) units, which can then be put together into long chains, called glycogen, which are then stored in the liver or muscles.

However, storage space is limited, and once it is full, the liver begins to convert excess glucose into fat. This process is called lipogenesis

Some of the newly created fat is stored in the liver, but most are transferred to other fat stores in the body. Although this is a more complex process, the amount of fat that can be created is unlimited.

So there are two complementary systems of food energy storage in the body. One is very easy to achieve but has limited storage capacity (glycogen), and the other is the more difficult to achieve but has unlimited storage capacity (body fat).

The process works in reverse when we don't eat (intermittent fasting). Insulin levels drop, signaling the body to start burning stored energy since it is no longer receiving any from food. Blood glucose drops, and the body must pull glucose from storage to burn it as energy. Glycogen is the most readily accessible source of energy. It breaks down into glucose molecules to provide energy to other cells. This can provide enough energy to the body for 24-36 hours. Then the body begins to break down fat to use as energy.

So the body can only be in two states: in an uptake state (high insulin) and a fasting state (low insulin). Either we are storing dietary energy or we are burning it. Either one or the other. If there is a balance between eating and fasting, there is no net weight gain.

If we start eating as soon as we get up and don't stop until we go to sleep, we spend most of our time in the absorption state. Over time, we will gain weight because we have not allowed the body time to burn off the stored energy.

To restore balance or lose weight, we just need to increase the interval in which we spend burning stored food energy.

This is intermittent fasting that allows the body to use stored energy.

If you eat consistently, every three hours, as is often recommended, your body will simply use the energy from the food that comes in. It may not need to burn much body fat if any at all. It will simply store it.

The body stores it for when there is nothing to eat.

If this happens it is because you lack balance. You lack intermittent fasting.

Chapter 3 :

Benefits Of Intermittent Fasting

The most obvious benefit of fasting is weight loss.

However, it has multiple benefits, many of which were well known in ancient times.

The fasting period is often referred to as a period of "cleansing" or "detoxification" by abstaining from food for a set period. People in the past thought that this period of abstinence from food would cleanse the body's systems of toxins and rejuvenate them. And it seems they were more right than they thought.

Some of the known physical benefits of fasting are:

⇒ Weight loss and body fat

⇒ Increased fat burning

⇒ Possible increase in energy

⇒ Decreased insulin and blood sugar levels

⇒ Possible reduction in inflammation

⇒ Possible correction of type 2 diabetes

⇒ Possible decrease in blood cholesterol

⇒ Possible improved alertness and concentration

⇒ Possible increase in growth hormone, at least in the short term

⇒ Possible life extension

⇒ Possible activation of cell cleansing by stimulating autophagy

Besides, fasting unlike many diets is free and not as expensive as dieting and often simplifies life and saves time for many people while diets take time away, while diets are limited concerning availability, fasting can be done anywhere.

The most effective diets for weight loss are those that are low in carbohydrates and high in fats. But also intermittent fasting gives its excellent results as the main focus is to reduce the effect of insulin. Many people believe that calories cause weight gain, this is simply a myth. Insulin is the main factor in weight gain. Low carbohydrate and high-fat diets lower insulin rather than calories but, intermittent fasting, is even better than a diet with the above principles, so you can combine the two for maximum effect.

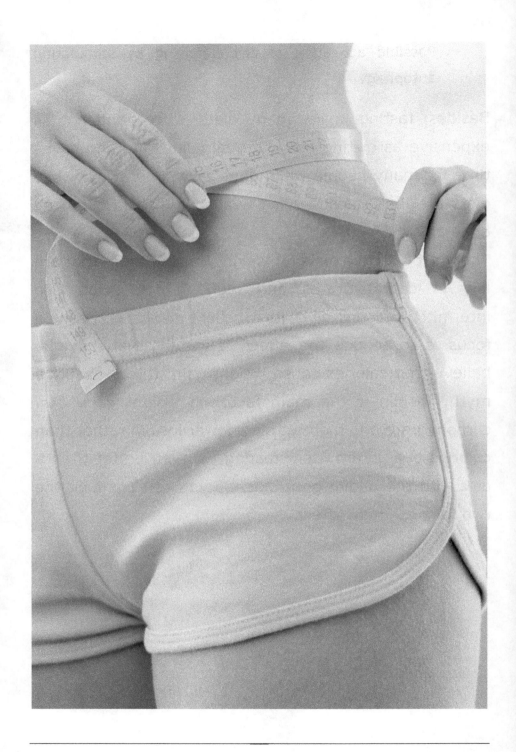

Chapter 4:

7 Advantages Of Intermittent Fasting

1: Flexibility

Fasting can be done anytime, anywhere. If for some reason you don't feel well, just stop. It is completely reversible in a matter of minutes.

There is no set duration. You can fast for 16 hours or 16 days. There is no set schedule. You can fast a lot this week and nothing next week. It can change according to your schedule. You can fast for any reason or no reason at all.

Also, why would we assume that a person can't fast for 1 week or 1 month without ever trying it?

2: Power

Losing weight is hard. And starting a diet with doubt that it will work is not among the most positive incentives. Often diets in which there's a reduction in calories don't work for everyone.

Some diets work amazingly for some people but fail for others. Sometimes diets work for some time and then seem to stagnate.

While intermittent fasting is effective having the fastest and most efficient way to lower insulin. Also, you have the option of "power" by continuing to fast until you reach your desired weight. The world record for fasting is 382 days, so it has unlimited power. So its effectiveness is unquestionable.

Fasting or low carb diet: Which is more powerful? Only two questions remain. The first: is it unhealthy? On the contrary, it has extraordinary health benefits. Second: can it be done? Well, if you never try it, you'll never know. I think almost anyone can do it.

3: It adds to any diet

This is the biggest benefit of all. Fasting can be added to any diet. This is because fasting is not something you do, but something you don't do. It is a subtraction rather than an addition.

If you were vegetarian, or gluten intolerant, or allergic to any food.... you can fast!

You don't have enough money to buy foods that fall into an "expensive" niche or you don't have time because you work and are away from home all day or you travel a lot or you don't like to cook...you can fast and feel informed, reach your ideal weight and feel good.

It's simple; it saves money; it saves time; it's flexible; it's effective; it can be done anytime, anywhere. What could be better than that?

4: Simplicity

People when they start a diet low in carbohydrates and high in fats do not need to understand what to eat and how it can give results. It is difficult to understand the differences between carbohydrates, fats, and proteins. Many foods contain hidden sugars in the ingredient list.

In the last 40-50 years people have always known that low-fat diets were the ones that brought results making it difficult for them to incorporate many natural healthy fats into their diet. A completely different approach like fasting was much easier for people to understand.

Fasting itself is so simple that it can be explained in two sentences. Don't eat anything, including sugar or sweeteners. Drink water, tea, coffee, or bone broth. That's it. Even with this simple method, understanding the details can take hours of explanation.

5: Economical

While I may prefer that patients eat organic, local meat and avoid white bread and processed foods, the truth is that these foods often cost 10 times as much. But not everyone unfortunately is allowed to eat that well so it's much cheaper to eat something with flour than with natural foods. This means that fresh cherries cost $6.99/pound and a whole loaf of bread costs $1.99. Feeding a family with little money is much easier by buying pasta and white bread.

 But that doesn't mean they are doomed to a lifetime of type 2 diabetes and disability. Fasting is free. It's not only free, but it saves you money because you don't have to buy food.

6: Convenience

Eating a homemade meal prepared from scratch is great, but many people simply don't have the time or inclination to do it. The amount of meals eaten outside the home has increased over the past few decades. .

 Don't get me wrong, I love to cook as much as the next person. But it takes a lot of time. Between work, writing, and family, I don't have a lot of time.

These days, we're all rushing around and doing a thousand things, and devoting time to cooking at home, as noble as it is, is not a winning strategy. On the other hand, fasting is the opposite. It saves time because you don't spend time buying food, preparing it, cooking it, or cleaning it. It's a way to simplify your life.

While many diets complicate your life (eat this, but not that, and just a little bit of the other), fasting simplifies it. Saving time and saving money? It doesn't get any better than that.

7: Cheat days

It's not practical to advise people to never eat ice cream again. Sure, you may be able to do without it for 6 months or 1 year, but a lifetime? And would you really want it? Think about it. Is it not possible to deprive ourselves of the pleasure of eating licorice forever?

You can't have dessert every day, but fasting gives you a chance to enjoy that dessert now and then because if you celebrate, you can balance the scales by fasting. This is, after all, the cycle of life. Celebration and fasting.

Simply put, following intermittent fasting makes following the diet easier and here it becomes a way of life. The most important aspect of fasting is fitting it into your life.

Life is intermittent. There are good days and bad days. There are days to celebrate and days to dread.... There are times when you eat a lot and celebrate, but equally, there must be days when you are restricted.

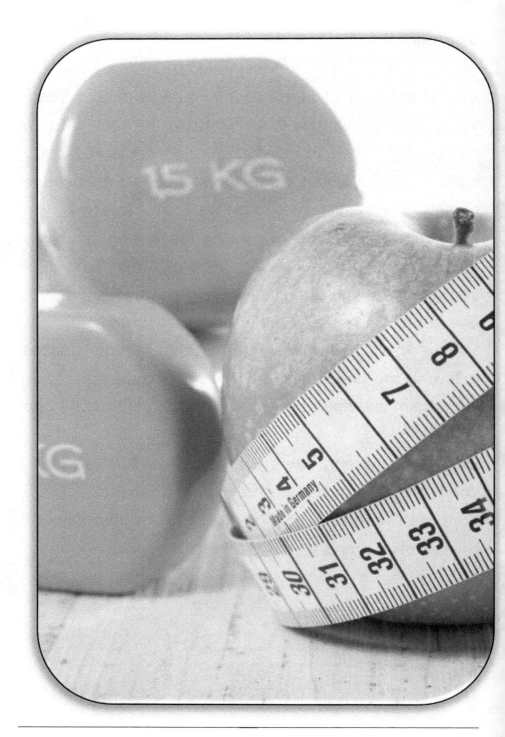

Chapter 5:

How to do intermittent fasting

People often ask if there are important differences between different fasting times, but the main difference, as you might suspect, is that shorter fasting periods are less effective and are usually done more frequently.

Therefore, the 16:8 fast is often done daily, while the 24-hour fast is done 2-3 times per week.

Much depends on how insulin resistant an individual is, in which case I prescribe the long fast and then follow up in the maintenance phase with shorter fasts.

The fasting protocol that best fits my lifestyle is to fast all day with a 4-5 hour interval between evening meals.

Fasting periods of less than 24 hours (20 hours fasting, 4 hours eating) can be done daily. The term "healthy" always depends on the goals you have. If you are simply trying to lose weight, then you can fast as needed to achieve it. There are no negative health consequences to eating only 4 hours a day.

However, it would be a good idea to change your fasting routine regularly, that way your body doesn't have a chance to adjust.

You have to find the routine that works best for you, however, physiologically, I think constantly changing things up works best.

The time of day you eat probably matters, but only a little. Mainly it depends on how it works best for you. It's best to try different times and see which works best for you, both from a lifestyle and weight loss standpoint. Deciding how long to continue fasting depends on what goals you set for yourself and how you feel. There is no set limit. Many people do a 1 week fast on their own or as part of a "cleanse".

Giving you personalized advice isn't easy and it wouldn't be fair the best thing to do is make your decision with your doctor.

Many people who approach this method of fasting at first are scared about how they feel the first few days. But again, it depends if you are a person who jumps right into doing things or prefer to do the steps slowly. It's your choice.

Short fasts (less than 24 hours)

Fasting offers quite a bit of flexibility. You can fast for as long as you want, but fasts that last longer than a couple of days may require medical supervision.

Shorter fasts are usually done more frequently.

16: 8

This form of intermittent fasting involves fasting, every day, for 16 hours. It is also sometimes called the 8-hour feeding window, or the 8-hour feeding window. All meals are eaten for 8 hours while fasting for the remaining 16 hours. This is usually done every day or nearly every day.

For example, you eat all meals between 11 a.m. and 7 p.m. This usually means skipping breakfast, although some people prefer to skip dinner. You usually eat two or three times during this 8-hour window.

20: 4

This is a 4-hour eating interval and a 20-hour fast. For example, you may eat between 2 and 6 p.m. each day and fast for the remaining 20 hours. This usually involves eating one or two small meals during this time interval.

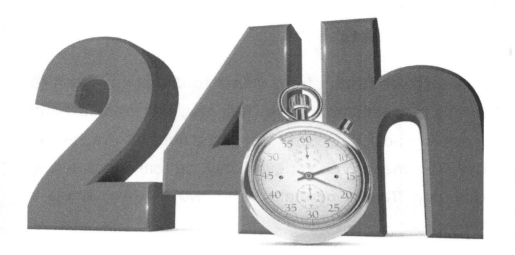

Long Fasts (24 hours or more)

24-Hour Fasts

This involves fasting from dinner to dinner (or lunch to lunch). You eat dinner on the first day, skip breakfast and lunch the next day, and return to dinner on the second day. This means you eat every day, but only once during that day. This is normally done two or three times a week.

Fasting 5:2

This is the version of intermittent fasting that has the most scientific support, as most studies on intermittent fasting have used similar practices.

It involves eating normally for 5 days and fasting for 2 days. However, 500 calories are allowed to be eaten during the fasting days. These calories can be consumed at any time, either spread throughout the day or in a single meal.

Every other day fasting

Another approach similar to 5:2 fasting is to have "fasting" days where you consume 500 calories, but instead of only doing it twice a week, you do it every other day.

36-hour fasts

You fast for an entire day. For example, if you eat dinner on the first day, you fast for the entire second day and don't eat again until breakfast on the third day. This is normally a 36-hour fast. This may provide additional weight loss benefits and may avoid the temptation to overeat on the second day.

Extended fasting

The first rule to keep in mind before doing longer fasts is to check with your doctor that you are not at risk of suffering complications. Usually, for fasts that last longer than 48 hours, it is recommended to take a multivitamin to avoid micronutrient deficiencies.

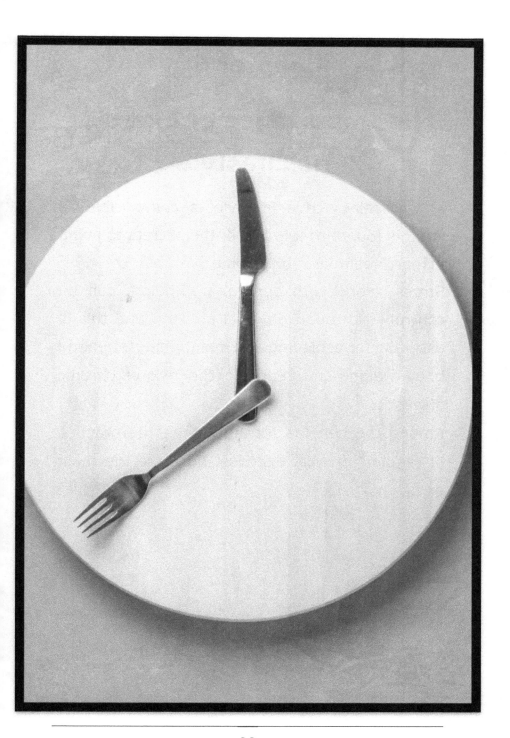

Chapter 6:

The Importance of Exercise as Lifestyle

A physically active lifestyle is comparable to youth's fountain: it is one of the secrets to living longer, healthier, and happier.

Stress, along with general well-being, can be controlled through physical activity, and this is essential for achieving and maintaining a healthy body weight and reducing the risk of chronic diseases.

Among the benefits attributable to the practice of regular physical exercise, here are the main ones:

- It reduces stress.

- It improves self-esteem, self-control, and a sense of general well-being.

- It helps you keep fit.

- It helps to strengthen bones, muscles, and joints.

- It increases muscle strength and endurance

- It allows to control the bodyweight.

- It reduces the risk of chronic diseases (vascular diseases, some cancers, type 2 diabetes mellitus).

- It improves the regulation of blood pressure in hypertensive and glycemic balance in diabetics.

- It reduces states of anxiety and depression.

Physical activity and nutrition are the two most important lifestyle variables for health. Staying active increases the amount of energy consumed, which is essential for weight control. As you age, your metabolism slows down, so you need to eat less and move more to keep your energy balance constant.

Implementation of Physical Activity

Incorporating into the daily routine of a constant and moderate physical activity induces a series of physiological changes in the organism that go beyond burning calories, reducing fat, and maintaining muscle mass. In addition to promoting weight loss and improving the relationship between food and the body itself, physical activity induces a change in the body's composition and the functioning of metabolism and systems (circulatory, respiratory, etc.)

Daily physical exercise, for example, is a way to improve cardiovascular health because it acts on different fronts:

- It reduces blood pressure, favoring the control of hypertension.

- It increases the secretion of HDL cholesterol (good cholesterol), reducing the rate of blood cholesterol.

- It induces a decrease in triglyceride levels.

- It decreases the production of insulin, helping to control type 2 diabetes, favoring the assimilation of nutrients, their arrival in the cells of the different tissues, and reducing the uptake and accumulation of fat.

Physical Activity

Control of cardiovascular risk factors (hypercholesterolemia, arterial hypertension, and type 2 diabetes).

- Increased lung capacity.

- Increase in muscle strength and mass.

- Increase in aerobic capacity.

- Reduction of fat mass.

It improves the person's psychological balance by inducing a state of personal satisfaction and the control of anxiety and stress.

Finally, it is worth highlighting the last benefit of physical activity. It improves the individual's relationship with food, reduces appetite, and favors the adoption of healthy eating habits.

We have to warn that in no way the IF approach can replace a direct health care provider, nor should it be used to determine a diagnosis, or to choose a procedure in particular cases.

What Are the best Types of Exercises for You (Woman Over 50)?

It is time to set the table, but the exercises from 50 should be to get a healthy body. The following exercises work several muscles in your body, as well as the buttocks and hamstrings for women over 50; create stronger legs, thinner and with more force, to lift your rear part, the quadriceps also work, since they require the knee to get resistance.

To perform the first of these exercises, stand in front of a bench or a firm chair and place your left foot firmly on top of the bench or chair. Press your left foot and push the body back until the left leg is straight; lower the body down until the right knee is flexed and repeat 10 to 15 times.

Weight balanced evenly; don't lean too far forward or too far back.

The so-called bridge exercises are not only the perfect exercise for a perfectly rounded back, but they will also help women keep their back healthy and pain-free.

Define Abs for Women

To do this great exercise called a bridge, lie down on the floor with your face up, with your knees slightly bent and with your feet flat on the floor. Raise your hips so that your body shapes will take a curved line from the shoulders to the knees. Pause in the upper position for two or three seconds, then lower your body back to the initial position. Repeat this movement 10 to 15 times; then take a short rest of five minutes maximum and repeat the number of times before recommended.

Routine Abdominals for Women

The addition of raising an arm while performing the previous exercise on the floor improves the posture and the strength of the base, which makes me feel better. It will seem more effort, but you will feel more secure.

Given the situation of reducing our belly, it is important to perform the exercises constantly and linearly; it is advisable to expand the abdominal table for women progressively. Every 10 or 15 days would be correct because each time we will have the most strengthened abdominal area.

Strengthen Buttocks

To perform the following exercise for women over 50 to create stronger, stronger legs and buttocks, start by adopting an iron position, but bend your elbows and lean on your forearms instead of on your hands.

Exercise Table for the Buttocks

Your body should create a straight line to the ankles from the shoulders.
Tighten your buttocks and maintain your hip position while raising your right arm forward;

move your shoulder blades down and back as you raise your arms. Keep the position for 5 to 10 seconds; relax the buttocks and repeat the exercise ten to fifteen times, alternating arms.

Yoga has so many physical and mental benefits. The postures are excellent to help reduce the appearance of cellulite. Make shoulder support or put your legs above the wall for 5 minutes every night before going to bed. This will be beneficial not only for the appearance of cellulite but also to collaborate greatly with leg circulation.

Exercises for Women Over 50 Years TO Create Stronger, Thinner, and Stronger Legs

To correctly perform the following exercise after 50, you have to take it more calmly.

To create stronger, more firm legs and buttocks, lie on your back and gradually lift your hips and legs off the floor, bringing your legs above your head until your toes touch the ground behind you.

Place your hands behind your back and extend your legs stretching them in the air, creating a straight line from your shoulders to your ankles. Keep your neck relaxed and your shoulder support hold, try to hold the position for at least one minute and then slowly reach the starting position, pause, rest, and then repeat the movement about ten more times, obviously with your respective breaks.

For a quick toning of the whole body, go through the movements described above and perform three sets of exercises about ten times or otherwise indicated by a medical condition; move as quickly as possible between the movements to the maximum calorie intake.

The next day, do other exercises. You can incorporate a few series of cardio intervals at the time of training your entire body; or you can do it separately over a longer period in these exercises for women over 50 years.

If you want to reinforce a specific part of your body, you should focus on exercises that train those particular muscles and incorporate them into your daily regimen. To continue to be effective, you should gradually increase the number of repetitions concerning how strong the muscle gets.

An Exercise Routine for Women Over 50

Multidirectional exercises help develop coordination and control while providing toning and hardening of the quadriceps, buttocks, hamstrings, and inner thighs.

Exercises after 50 Will Help Keep Your Back Healthy and Pain-Free

To perform the following exercise, stand with your feet together, both arms stretched over your head, palms facing foward.

Take a wide step with your right foot towards the corner of the room at a 45-degree angle and diagonally, bending the right knee and reaching the lower part of your body in a forward motion on your right thigh.

The back leg should be straight, with your heel lifted off the floor.

Leg and Buttock Exercises

If you can touch the ground, do it on both sides of your right foot, lightly with your fingers. Push with your right foot to return to the starting position.

Repeat 15 times on one leg and 15 times for the other. An option to modify this exercise is not to go so low in the stride and aim to reach with your hands at the knee or the level of the shin instead.

Leg Exercises for Women

As quick advice, stand again out of the position described above and focus on working out the abdominals with tight buttocks, squeezing your thighs together, and maintaining good posture. In addition to getting thinner and stronger legs, the postures that we must adapt maintain a healthy and erect back. In addition to hardening our legs, our day to day will have a better quality of life. Now I remember what it cost to climb the stairs with a smile from ear to ear.

Chapter 7:

What Is the Omad Diet

OMAD stands for "one meal a day" It is a form of intermittent fasting. This menu helps you prepare OMAD safely and effectively, with enough calories and protein, to help you reach your weight loss and low-carb goals.

The OMAD diet is the longest form of a limited-time window diet, equivalent to a 23: 1 fast (23 hours of fasting and ability to eat in a 1-hour time window). In its purest form, the OMAD diet does not impose a specific caloric restriction or macronutrient composition. As such, we recommend continuing the healthy low-carb diet during that meal.

Is OMAD Good for Weight Loss?

When the body is in a fasting state, it uses fat reserves as fuel for energy. This leads to the breakdown and utilization of fat, which helps in maintaining lifestyle-related disorders. It also reduces inflammation levels and increases growth hormone (HGH) levels that help burn fat.

Consumption of fibrous fruits and vegetables leads to less absorption of sugar and fat in the body. Fiber also improves digestion and relieves constipation. All of these characteristics lead collectively to weight reduction.

Advantages of the OMAD Diet:

⇒ OMAD diet leads to weight loss: Intermittent fasting and only 1 meal per day reduce caloric intake thus promoting weight loss.

⇒ Useful in type II diabetes: Intake of fiber-rich foods with low glycemic index controls blood sugar spikes. Weight reduction also helps reduce hyperinsulinemia.

⇒ Heart-friendly: Reduces visceral fat and improves heart function.

⇒ Feeling light: Intermittent fasting reduces fat deposits in the body, making you more active and less fatigued.

⇒ Assistant for self-control: The OMAD diet inculcates the habit of selecting nutritious foods. Consciously, with practice, you will overcome your cravings and overeating.

Many of those who eat an OMAD model tend to do so just for the ease of preparing food and eating once a day. This can be especially helpful for those who travel frequently, those on shifts at work, and those with busy, hectic schedules.

Think about how much time you spend shopping, planning, and preparing meals. (And let's not even talk about dirty dishes). If there are three meals a day, how much time could you save by cutting out two-thirds?

Some people see the OMAD diet as an "easy" way to reduce calorie intake. When eating is only allowed in a 30-60 minutes time period, it becomes physically difficult to exceed your daily calorie requirements.

OMAD Diet Side Effects:

- Overeating or bingeing: When you start with OMAD, fasting for 23 hours may cause you to choose unhealthy food options. You get uncontrollable cravings for junk food and desserts. This gets better with time. As your body begins to accept the routine.

- Hypoglycemia: There is always a risk of a lack of energy. In severe cases, the person may go dark. Other symptoms include constant hunger, fatigue, shaking, inability to concentrate, and irritability. This also improves with time.

- Consistency: Calorie restriction will initially cause weight loss. But it is difficult to stick to this routine on a permanent basis. So, this may lead to weight recycling.

- Physical and Psychological Symptoms: Intermittent fasting increases stress on the body leading to anxiety-related disorders like nausea and mouth ulcers. Acidity can become a problem if your other lifestyle traits are not correct. For instance, improper sleep and OMAD in combination can lead to acidity and reflux together.

- Sleep Disorder: Intermittent fasting and calorie restriction could affect the central nervous system. This may affect the clarity, focus, and rhythm of sleep.

- Difficult to follow: It takes willpower and fortitude to stick to this diet pattern.

OMAD is definitely not a good option for those who lack motivation and cannot resist temptation.

Chapter 8:

Foods to Include in the Omad Diet and to Avoid:

You Can Include

⇒ Vegetables: Green leafy vegetables, carrot, broccoli, cabbage, cauliflower, red beet, lettuce, bell peppers, sweet potatoes, and squash.

⇒ Fruits: Apple, banana, orange, grapefruit, grapes, cucumber, tomato, peach, plum, lemon, lime, pineapple, and berries.

⇒ Animal protein: White meat such as chicken, lean meat, fish, and eggs.

⇒ Vegetable proteins: Legumes, dal, mushrooms, soybeans, tofu, nuts, and seeds.

⇒ Milk and its products: Whole milk, curds, cheese, buttermilk, and paneer.

⇒ Whole grains: Brown rice, black rice, cracked wheat, millet, quinoa, and barley.

⇒ Fats and oils: Omega-3-rich olive oil, MUFA-rich rice bran oil, sunflower butter, peanut butter, coconut oil, and almond butter.

⇒ Nut and Seeds: MUFA- and PUFA-rich nuts such as almonds, walnuts, pistachios, sunflower seeds, pumpkin seeds, and melon seeds.

⇒ Herbs and Spices: Mint, fennel, thyme, oregano, garlic, ginger, onion, coriander, cumin, turmeric, pepper, cardamom, and cloves.

⇒ Beverages: Zero-calorie beverages such as water, homemade salted lemonade, green tea, black tea, or sugar-free black coffee.

You Cannot Include

⇒ Fruits Consume: Grapes, Jackfruit, Mango, Chikoo, Sitaphal and Pineapple in very small amounts.

⇒ Canned foods: Canned meats, pineapples, cherries, jams, jellies or olives as it contains many preservatives, sugar, and salt.

⇒ Milk and its products: Low-fat milk and products, flavored yogurt and cream cheese.

⇒ Grains: with a high glycemic index such as rice and refined flour as they could lead to weight gain.

⇒ Nuts and seeds: Limit consumption of cashews as it could also lead to weight gain.

⇒ Fats and oils: Trans fats containing margarine, lard, vegetable oil, butter, and mayonnaise to prevent heart disease.

⇒ Beverages: Packaged fruit and vegetable juices, carbonated drinks and energy drinks as they contain simple sugars that lead to weight gain.

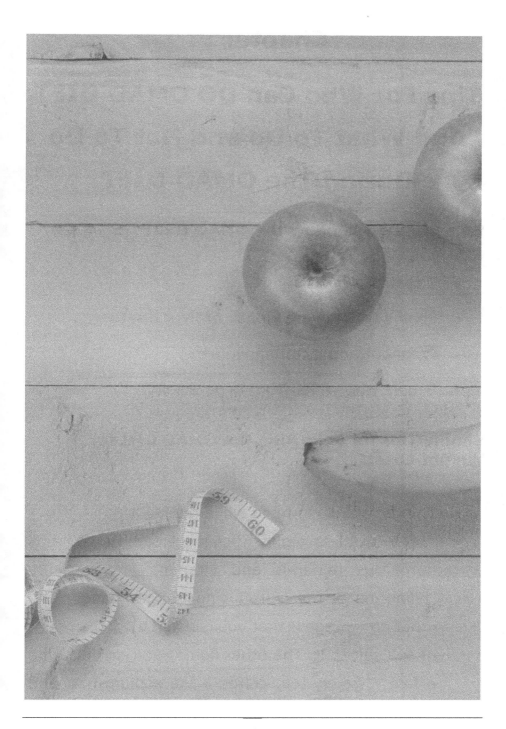

Chapter 9:

Tips For Who Can DO OMAD DIET And What To Do and Not To Do During The OMAD DIET

Who Shouldn't Follow the OMAD Diet?

- Diabetics on insulin.

- People with severe kidney or liver disease.

- Pregnant and lactating women.

- People who suffer from hyperacidity.

Simple Tips for Following the OMAD Diet for Weight Loss:

- Things to keep in mind while fasting are:

- Bone broth is highly recommended. It contains numerous minerals and vitamins and is quite "filling" in terms of reducing hunger pangs. The other advantage is that you can add a good amount of sea salt to it. The other liquids you drink during a fast - water, tea, coffee - are sodium-free and can lead to dehydration. Mild dehydration, for example, can lead to cramps and headaches during a longer fast.

- So yes, bone broth is highly recommended. Also, it is a very traditional food with ancient healing traditions.

- You can drink other liquids during the fast such as tea (all kinds, including mate), coffee is all acceptable. And why not even a small amount of cream or coconut oil in the coffee for better adhesion, although technically it would not be allowed and possible to do so.

- Keep yourself sufficiently hydrated.

- Start by following the pattern for 1-2 days a week.

- Gradually increase the number of days until you feel comfortable.

- You can choose the mealtime according to your convenience.

- It is important to eat at the same time every day.

- You can consume 3-4 cups of zero-calorie green tea or spiced teas during the fasting phase.

- Consume an egg or 1 serving of nuts before working out.

- Drink coconut water after your workout to replace electrolytes.

- Get at least 7 to 8 hours of sleep.

- Avoid junk foods and fruit juices.

To Finish about OMAD

The OMAD diet is effective in weight loss and prevents weight regain. But every individual will react differently to this program. It will only work wonders if you choose healthy lifestyle. Always consult a qualified professional before trying anything new. The best path to a sustainable life is through a healthy and balanced diet, regular exercise, and a healthy lifestyle.

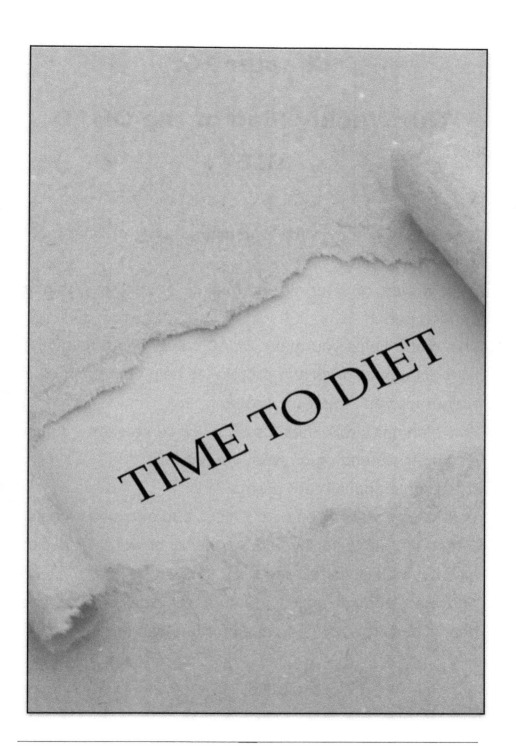

Chapter 10:

The Weekly Plan of the OMAD DIET

OMAD is an acronym for "one meal a day", or "one meal a day" in Spanish.

It is a way of intermittent fasting or eating within a defined period.

This menu helps you make OMAD safely and effectively, with enough calories and protein, to help you reach your weight loss and low-carb goals.

This plan has single meal days, which can be either lunch or dinner depending on what you prefer.

It is simple and without drama.

In addition, you will enjoy delicious and nutritious meals.

Of course, make sure you drink plenty of water (you can also have black coffee and tea).

And eat enough salt to minimize side effects like headaches. The recipes are all for one serving

Easy Keto Bacon and Eggs Dish

Monday Meal

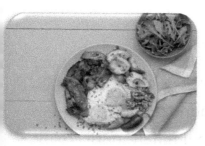

Time 5 + 10 m | beginner

Don't be shy and enjoy this classic keto breakfast for lunch or dinner. We have added walnuts and peppers to make it crisp. Why complicate things?

Ingredients:

- 2 1/2 oz. smoked bacon

- 2 eggs

- 1 (7 oz.) avocados

- 2 tbsp. walnuts

- ½ (2 ½ oz.) green bell peppers

- Salt and ground black pepper

- ½ tbsp. fresh chives,finely,cho pped

At your service:

¼ cup rocket salad and ½ tbsp. olive oil

Instructions:

The steps to follow are written for 1 serving. Take this into account if you are preparing more servings.

1. Fry the bacon in butter over medium heat until crispy.

2. Remove from the pan and keep warm. Leave the accumulated fat in the pan. Lower the heat to medium-low and fry the eggs in the same skillet.

3. Place the bacon, eggs, avocado, walnuts, bell pepper and rocket salad on a plate.

4. Pour the remaining bacon fat over the eggs. Season to taste.

   Low carb ketogenic (kcal: 937 - We do not recommend counting calories.)

Per portion:

- Net carbs: 4% (9 g)
- Fat: 78% (78 g)

- Fiber: 16 g
- Protein: 19% (42 g)

The Classic Keto Cheeseburger

Tuesday Meal

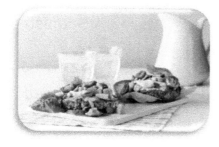

Time 20 + 15 m |
medium   difficulty

Cheeseburgers ... Can there be a better entree for a keto feast? They taste good and fill you up, but they are made effortlessly! And you don't need to put them on bread to dress them with delicious Mexican sauce!

Sauce Ingredients:

- ½ (1.94 oz.) tomatoes

- ½ (0.26 oz.) chives

- ¼ (1.76 oz.) avocados

- ¼ tbsp. olive oil

- ½ tbsp. chopped fresh cilantro

- Salt to taste

Burgers Ingredients:

- 6 oz. ground beef (minced meat)

- ¼ cup (1 oz.) grated cheddar cheese, divided into two parts

- ½ tsp. garlic powder

- ½ tsp. onion powder

- ½ tsp. Spanish paprika

- ½ tsp. finely chopped fresh oregano

- ½ tbsp. butter, for frying

Toppings:

1 ¼ oz. romaine lettuce

2 tbsp. mayonnaise

1 ¼ cooked smoked bacon, crumbled

1 tbsp. chopped pickled jalapeños

0.63 oz. pickled gherkins, sliced

1 tbsp. Dijon mustard

Instructions:

The steps to follow are written for 1 serving. Take this into account if you are preparing more servings.

1. Chop the sauce ingredients and stir well in a small bowl. Reserve.

2. Mix the seasonings and half of the cheese with the ground beef.

3. Assemble four hamburgers and fry them in a pan or on a grill if you prefer. Add the remaining cheese on top towards the end.

4. Serve on lettuce leaves with pickles and mustard. On top, place the bacon. And don't forget about the homemade Mexican salsa!

Low carb ketogenic (kcal: 1007 - We do not recommend counting calories.)

Per portion:

- Net carbs: 3% (8 g)

- Fiber: 7 g

- Fat: 75% (82 g)

- Protein: 22% (55 g)

Keto Tuna Dish

Wednesday Meal

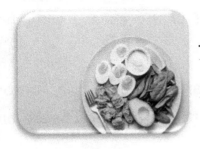

Time 5 + 10 m |

beginner

Real food on a plate. Tuna, eggs, spinach, avocado, mayonnaise, and lemon. Because a keto meal doesn't have to be complicated.

Ingredients:

- 2 eggs

- 1 oz.(1 cup) spinach sprouts

- 5 oz. tuna in olive oil

- ½ (3 ½ oz.) avocados

- ¼ cup mayonnaise

- 1/8 lemon (optional)

- salt - pepper to taste

Instructions:

The steps to follow are written for 1 serving. Take this into account if you are preparing more servings.

1. Start by cooking the eggs. Add them carefully to boiling water and cook them for 4-8 minutes, depending on whether you like them poached or hard.

2. Chill the eggs in ice water for 1-2 minutes when done; this will make it easier to peel them off.

3. Place the eggs, spinach, tuna and avocado on a plate. Serve with a good dollop of mayonnaise and a lemon wedge if you feel like it. Season to taste.

Low carb ketogenic (kcal: 930 - We do not recommend counting calories.)

Per portion:

- Net carbs: 1% (3 g)

- Fiber: 7 g

- Fat: 76% (76 g)

- Protein: 23% (52 g)

Keto Italian Chicken with Cabbage Pasta

Thursday Meal

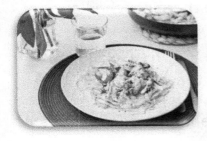

Time 15 + 30 m |
medium difficulty

A simple and creamy dinner. Chicken, Parmesan cheese, and the tangy touch of sun-dried tomatoes. It serves you as a normal weeknight dinner or for a weekend with friends. Serve alongside butter-fried cabbage strips instead of pasta. One more success of the keto kitchen!

Ingredients:

- ½ tbsp. butter for frying

- 6 oz. boneless chicken drumsticks, sliced

- 1 tbsp. dried tomatoes in oil, finely chopped

- 2 cherry tomatoes cut into four pieces

- ¼ garlic cloves, finely minced

- ¼ cream (or cream) to whip

- 1/3 cup grated Parmesan cheese

- ¼ cup spinach sprouts

- salt and pepper

Cabbage paste:

- 2.82 oz. shredded white cabbage
- ½ tbsp. butter for frying salt or pepper

Instructions:

The steps to follow are written for 1 serving. Take this into account if you are preparing more servings.

1. Heat the butter in a skillet over medium heat. Fry the chicken for a couple of minutes. In this instance it is not necessary to cook it completely, since then it will continue cooking with the next ingredients. Salt and pepper.

2. Add the two types of tomatoes to the pan, along with the garlic.

3. Add the whipping cream. Let it boil over medium heat for about 5 minutes.

4. Add the grated Parmesan cheese and simmer for another 10 minutes. Season to taste.

5. Meanwhile, melt the butter over medium heat in a large skillet. Add the cabbage and fry until tender. Season to taste.

6. Spread the cabbage on serving plates. Add the spinach to the pan with the creamy chicken and stir. Finally, pour the chicken along with the creamy sauce on top of the cabbage.

Tips:

- Chicken Parmesan goes great with cauliflower rice. If you want to discover more of our garnishes, here they are all.

- You can substitute the spinach for chopped kale (without the stems).

Moderate low-Carb (kcal: 653 - We do not recommend counting calories.)

Per portion

- Net carbs: 5% (8g)

- Fiber: 3 g

- Protein: 29%(46g) / Fat: 66% (48g)

Ketogenic Fat Head Pizza

Friday Meal

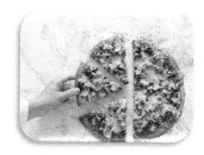

Time: 15 + 30 m | Moderate

You can add all your favorite toppings to this crispy, keto, cheese-laden pizza crust that is really going to nourish and fill you up. Bon Appetite!

Ingredients base:

- ¾ cup (3 oz.) grated mozzarella cheese

- 6 tbsp. (1 ½ oz.) almond flour

- 1 tbsp. cream cheese

- 1/2 tsp. white wine vinegar

- ½ egg

- ¼ tsp. salt

- Olive oil to grease the hands

Ingredients on the base:

- 4 oz. Italian sausages

- ½ tbsp. butter

- ¼ cup tomato sauce without sugar

- ¼ tsp. dried oregano
- ¾ cup (3 oz.) mozzarella cheese

Instructions:

Instructions are for 1 serving. Modify them as needed

1. Preheat the oven to 200 ° C (400 ° F).

2. Heat the mozzarella and cream cheese in a small nonstick pot over medium heat or in a bowl in the microwave.

3. Mix until the mozzarella and cream cheese are melted and incorporated. Add the other ingredients and mix well.

4. Moisten your hands with olive oil and flatten the dough on parchment paper to form a circle about 20 cm (8 inches) in diameter. You can also use a rolling pin to flatten the dough between two sheets of parchment paper.

5. Remove the top sheet of parchment paper (if you used it). Prick the dough with a fork (all over the surface) and bake for 10-12 minutes until golden brown. Take out of the oven.

6. While the dough is baking, sauté the ground sausage in olive oil or butter.

7. Spread a thin layer of tomato sauce over the dough. Top with the pork and plenty of cheese. Bake for 10-15 more or until cheese has melted.

8. Sprinkle oregano on top and serve with a green salad.

Advice!

Bake additional batter and freeze for a quick and easy dinner. Or, use the extra batter to make a Rosemary Garlic Focaccia Bread-just sprinkle garlic butter on top and bake for another couple of minutes.

Low carb ketogenic (kcal: 1235 - We do not recommend counting calories.)

Half a pizza:

Net carbs: 4% (13 g)

Fiber: 1 g

Fat: 74% (100 g)

Protein: 22% (66 g)

Keto Chicken Wings with Creamy Broccoli

Saturday Meal

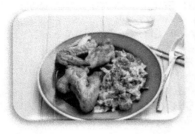

Time 10 + 45 m | Easy

With this simple dish, you will win over the whole world! These tender chicken wings taste like glory. Combined with the creamy broccoli they are great for weeknight dinner.

Ingredients Grilled chicken wings:

- 11.46 oz. chicken wings

- 1/8 orange, juice and zest

- 1 tbsp. olive oil

- ½ tsp. powdered ginger

- ¼ tsp. salt

- 1/10 tsp. cayenne pepper

Creamy broccoli:

- 6 oz. broccoli

- ¼ cup mayonnaise

- 1 tbsp. (1/50 oz.) chopped fresh dill

- salt and pepper to taste

Instructions:

Instructions are for 1 serving. Modify them as needed.

1. Preheat the oven to 200 °C (400 °F).

2. Mix the orange juice and zest with the oil and spices in a small bowl. Place the chicken wings in a plastic bag and add the marinade.

3. Shake the bag well so that the wings are well bathed in the mixture. Let marinate for at least 5 minutes. If possible, allow a little more time.

4. Arrange the wings in a single layer on a greased roasting pan.

5. Bake on a wire rack in the middle of the oven for about 45 minutes or until the wings are golden brown and well done.

6. Meanwhile, cut the broccoli into small florets and boil in salted water for a couple of minutes. They should only soften a bit, without losing their shape or color.

7. Strain the broccoli and let some of the steam evaporate. Mix with the mayonnaise and dill. Season to taste.

8. Serve the broccoli along with the roasted wings.

Advice!

You can substitute broccoli for small florets of cauliflower or Brussels sprouts. If you have an outdoor grill, you can also use it to cook your wings

Low carb ketogenic (kcal: 1216 - We do not recommend counting calories.)

Per portion:

- Net Carbs: 3%(9g)

- Fiber: 5 g

- Fat: 75% (99 g)

- Protein: 22%(65 g)

Keto Herb Butter Cheese Steak Roulades

Sunday Meal

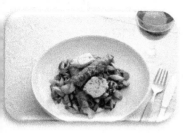

Time 10 + 20 m |

Moderate

This is quite a keto delicacy. Tasty meat stuffed with cheese and served over leeks and mushrooms. A marvel for any night. And don't forget the herb butter, it adds a lot of aromas.

Ingredients:

- ½ (1 ½ oz.) leek

- 3.88 oz.mushrooms

- Two thin steaks

- ½ tbsp. olive oil

- salt and pepper

- 0.74 oz.   (3 tbsp.) cheddar cheese or gruyere cheese

- Two chopsticks

- ½ tbsp. butter for frying

- 1 ¼ oz. butter with herbs

Instructions:

The steps to follow are written for 1 serving. Take this into account if you are preparing more servings.

1. Trim and rinse the leeks. Cut into wide slices, using the white and green parts. Cut the mushrooms into pieces.

2. Fry the mushrooms and leeks in olive oil until they take on a good color. Season to taste. Place in a bowl and cover to keep everything warm.

3. Place the thin steaks on a large cutting board. Season to taste. Place a stick of cheese on each steak and roll. Close with a toothpick.

4. Sauté the roulades over medium heat for 10-15 minutes and reduce heat towards the end.

5. Pour the juices over the leeks and mushrooms. Serve the roulades with herb butter and the fried vegetables. Don't forget to remove the toothpick before serving!

Advice!

You can also add a pinch of chili flakes to give the leeks a spicy touch.

Low carb ketogenic (kcal: 726 - We do not recommend counting calories.)

Per portion:

- Net Carbs:3%(5g

- Fiber: 2 g

- Fat: 73% (59 g)

- Protein: 24% (44 g)

Chapter 11:

OMAD Diet Weekly Plan with Snack

In this week I suggest that if you are not yet 100% ready to eat once a day that you have a snack 30 minutes before the main meal 3 days a week.

As a snack you will eat in those days, the leftovers of the dinner of the previous day try to stick to 16: 8 intermittent fasting in these days. While for the rest you will adopt one meal per day. The recipes are all for one serving.

Keto cheese rolls
Monday Meal

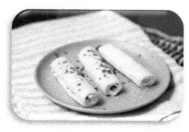

Time: 5m | easy

This is the fastest, simplest, and tastiest keto recipe in the world. It's impossible to resist this salty treat! Ideal for a snack.

Ingredients

2 oz. (½ cup) sliced cheddar or provolone cheese or edam cheese

- ½ oz. Butter

Instructions

1. Place the cheese slices on a large cutting board.

2. Thinly slice the butter using a cheese slicer or knife.

3. Cover each slice of cheese with butter and roll up. Serve as a breakfast or snack.

Advice

These cheese rolls are delicious as is, but you can also add a few extras. For example, it combines wonderfully with powdered paprika, salt flakes, parsley, or other finely chopped herbs

Keto pork chops with blue cheese sauce
Tuesday Meal

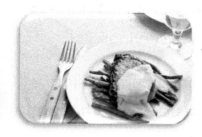

Time 5 + 15 m | easy

Salty and flavorful, this blue cheese dip dresses up any chop - and figuratively leads it to dance - in this incredibly simple and delicious meal. Light the fire and let the show begin!

Ingredients

- 1 ¼ oz. blue cheese

- 3 tbsp. whipping cream or heavy cream

- 1 pork chops

- 1 ¾ oz. fresh green beans (green beans)

- ½ tbsp. butter for frying

- salt and pepper

Instructions

The steps to follow are written for 4 servings. Take this into account if you are preparing fewer servings.

1. Start by crushing the cheese and pouring it into a small saucepan over medium heat. Adjust the heat as needed so that it melts gently being careful not to let it burn. When the cheese has melted, add the cream or fresh cream and increase the heat a little. Let it simmer for a few minutes.

2. Season the chops. Fry them in a skillet over medium-high heat for 2-3 minutes before turning. Cook until the internal temperature is 63-71 C ° (145 ° -160 ° F). Reserve and cover with aluminum foil for 2-3 minutes.

3. Pour the juices from the pan into the cheese sauce. Stir and, if necessary, raise the heat again. Since blue cheese is usually quite salty, taste the sauce before adding more salt.

4. Trim and clarify the green beans. Fry them in butter for a few minutes over medium heat. Salt and pepper

Low carb broccoli and cheese
Wednesday Meal

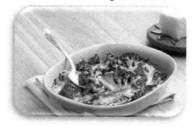

Time 5 + 15 m | easy

Classic Broccoli Wisdom - Kids will ask to repeat if your recipe includes a lot of butter and cheese! Sign up for a delicious, melt-in-your-mouth taste of serving this tried-and-true side dish.

Ingredients

¼ lb broccoli

$^4/_5$ oz. Butter

salt and ground black pepper

¼ oz. (5 tbsp) cheddar cheese, grated

Instructions

The steps to follow are written for 4 servings. Take this into account if you are preparing fewer servings.

1. Preheat the oven to 200 ° C (400 ° F). Or, better yet, put the grill to the maximum

2. Divide the broccoli into buds and boil in slightly salted water for a few minutes. Make sure the broccoli retains its crisp texture and fresh green color.

3. Drain all the liquid and place the cooked broccoli in a well greased baking dish. Add the butter and pepper and salt.

4. Sprinkle the cheese over the broccoli and bake for 15-20 minutes until the cheese begins to brown. If you use the grill, this step may be faster. Take a look at the term and take it out when the cheese starts to brown.

Keto Italian meatballs

Thursday Meal

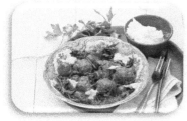

Time 10 + 45 m | medium difficulty

Meatballs: with just the right touch of onion and oregano. Tomato sauce: rich and comforting. Mozzarella: fresh and creamy. Every bite of this recipe: Delicious

Ingredients

¼ lb ground beef (minced meat)

½ oz. grated

Parmesan cheese

¼ egg

$1 / 8$ tbsp. dried basil

$1 / 8$ tsp. onion powder

½ tbsp. fresh parsley, finely chopped

¼ tsp. garlic powder

¼ tsp. Salt

$1 / 8$ tsp. ground black pepper

¾ tbsp. olive oil

3 ½ oz. (6 $2 / 3$ tbsp.) canned whole tomatoes

1 ¾ oz. fresh spinach

½ oz. Butter

1 ¼ oz. mozzarella cheese balls or mozzarella cheese

salt and ground black pepper

Instructions

1. Place the ground beef, Parmesan cheese, eggs, salt, and spices in a bowl and mix well. With the mixture, make meatballs of approximately 30 grams (1 ounce) each. To make the process easier, we recommend keeping your hands moist while the meatballs are assembling
2. In a skillet, heat the olive oil and sauté the meatballs until golden brown on all sides
3. Lower the heat and add the canned tomatoes. Let simmer for 15 minutes, stirring every couple of minutes. Season to taste. Add the parsley and stir. If you want to freeze the dish, this would be the last stage

4. In another pan, melt the butter and fry the spinach for 1-2 minutes, stirring continuously. Season to taste. Add the spinach to the meatballs. Top with fresh mozzarella cheese, cut into bite-size pieces. Serve and enjoy.

Keto three cheese omelette
Friday Meal

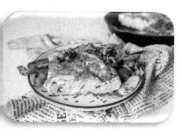

Time 20 + 20 m | easy

Creamy cheese on the inside and crispy bacon on top, who cannot love this simple and delicious omelet? It is perfect for breakfast, brunch, lunch or dinner. Surprise your family and friends with this elegant dish accompanied by a salad

Ingredients

½ tbsp. ghee or melted butter

2 eggs

3 tbsp. cream to whip

¼ cup ricotta cheese

¼ cup (1 oz.) Shredded cheddar cheese

½ oz. feta cheese

3 oz. smoked bacon, fried and cut into small pieces

2 tbsp. fresh spinach, finely chunked

Instructions

1. Grease a 12 "(30 cm) skillet with butter or ghee
2. In a large bowl, whisk together the eggs, cream, salt, and pepper
3. Pour the egg mixture into the skillet and put it over medium heat.
4. Sprinkle the grated cheddar cheese over the eggs, also add the ricotta cheese and crumbled feta cheese
5. Add the spinach and bacon pieces to the egg mixture and stir gently.
6. Preheat the top rack or oven rack. When the edges of the tortilla begin to set on the top rack, in about 10 minutes, place the pan under the grill to finish it.

7. The tortilla will be done when the center is cooked and golden on top

Advice

Be careful how much salt you add as feta cheese is usually quite salty. Taste the feta cheese first and adjust the amount of salt.

Serve the hot omelet with very crispy bacon and a green salad.

To make a simple salad dressing, drizzle some hot bacon fat over your veggies and toss it with a splash of apple cider vinegar

Keto Kale Warm Salad
Saturday Meal

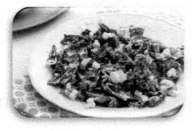

Time 10 + 10 m | easy

Sautéed kale takes the lead in this fabulous, crunchy keto salad. Together, the delicious blue cheese, Dijon mustard and garlic will be a hit. They deserve a standing ovation. It is fabulous as a garnish with almost any meal.

Ingredients

butter½ oz.

55 g kale

salt and ground black pepper

45 ml cream (or cream) to whip

½ tbsp. Mayonnaise

¼ tsp. Dijon mustard

½ tbsp. olive oil

¼ garlic cloves, minced or minced

28 g blue cheese or

feta cheese

Instructions

1. Combine the heavy cream, mayonnaise, mustard, olive oil, and garlic in a small measuring glass. Season to taste.
2. Rinse the kale and cut into small, bite-sized pieces. Remove and throw away the thick stem
3. Heat a large skillet and add the butter. Sauté the kale quickly for a nice color, but no more. Season to taste.
4. Place in a salad bowl and pour the dressing on top. Stir well and serve with crumbled blue
5. cheese or some other tasty cheese

Keto tri-color roasted veggie chicken
Sunday Meal

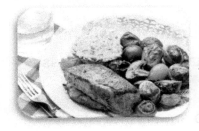

Time 15 + 30 m | easy

A quick and simple meal does not have to skimp on quality or quantity. This fried chicken along with a classic and colorful trio of vegetables is not only prepared in the blink of an eye, it is also very satiating. Your belly will thank you

Ingredients

Tricolor roasted vegetables

¼ lb Brussels sprouts

2 oz. cherry tomatoes

¼ tsp. dried rosemary

2 oz. mushrooms

¼ tsp. sea salt

$1/8$ tsp. ground black pepper

2 tbsp. olive oil

Fried chicken

1 (10 oz.) chicken
breasts (skinless)

¼ oz. butter, for frying

1 oz. herbed
butter, for serving

Instructions

1. Preheat the oven to 200 ° C (400 ° F). Place the whole vegetables in a roasting pan

2. Add salt, pepper and rosemary. Pour olive oil on top and stir so that it mixes with the vegetables evenly

3. Bake for 20 minutes or until vegetables are lightly caramelized

4. Meanwhile, fry the chicken in olive oil or butter and season. Cook until a meat thermometer inserted into the largest piece shows 165 ° F (74 ° C).

Keto queen avocado
Extra recipe for meal replacement

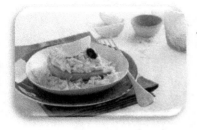 Time 120 + 20 m | easy

Who doesn't like avocado? This tasty Chilean dish is a complete meal that is easy to make and combines a few favorite ingredients.

Ingredients

5 ⅓ oz. small chicken breasts (without skin)

2/5 tsp. salt, or to taste, divided

$1/8$ tsp. freshly ground pepper, or to taste, divided

½ tbsp. avocado oil

$1/10$ cup avocado oil

¼ tsp. Dijon mustard

⅔ oz. red bell peppers, minced

At your service

½ (3 ½ oz.) Avocados big

¼ green lemons, juiced

½ oz. iceberg lettuce, cut into strips

¼ tbsp. avocado oil

$1/8$ tsp. Salt

¼ hard-boiled egg,
quartered

1 black olives

1/10 tsp. freshly
ground pepper, or
to taste

Instructions

1. Season the breasts with a teaspoon of salt and a pinch of pepper
2. Heat the avocado oil in a skillet over medium-high heat
3. Fry the breasts until they are golden brown on the bottom
4. Flip and cook other side in the same way, or until meat marks 165 ° F (75 ° C) in the middle, measured with a meat thermometer
5. Remove from heat and allow to cool to room temperature
6. When the chicken has cooled, shred it with a fork
7. Mix the chicken with the mayonnaise, the mustard and the chopped pepper. Season with salt and pepper to taste
8. Chill in the refrigerator for a couple of hours.

At your service

1. Peel the avocados and remove the seed. Spread the avocados with the lemon juice.

2. Place the lettuce on the serving plate, pour the oil over the lettuce and season with a little salt. Place the avocados on the lettuce and fill these with the chicken.

3. Garnish each avocado with a quarter egg and an olive. Sprinkle with pepper to taste.

Keto pizza-style omelet
Extra recipe for meal replacement

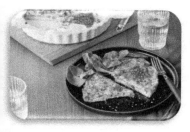

Time 10 + 30 m | easy

Is it an omelet? A pizza? Or maybe a quiche? It doesn't matter! If it tastes this good and is also keto, call it what you want. Just be sure to invite all of your friends to share this simple and delicious dinner

Ingredients Mass

2 eggs

2 ⅔ oz. mozzarella cheese

1 oz. cream cheese

1 / 8 tsp. Salt

½ tsp. garlic powder (optional)

Stuffed

1 ½ tbsp. ketchup

3 oz. grated mozzarella cheese

1 tsp. Dried oregano

Instructions

1. Preheat the oven to 200 ° C (400 ° F)
2. Start by making the dough. Break the eggs into a medium bowl and incorporate the rest of the ingredients. Stir well to combine everything
3. Line a cake pan (a normal cake pan is big enough for two servings), or any other oven-safe dish with parchment paper (crease the paper before flattening it so it stays down more easily). Pour the pizza dough. Spread it evenly with a spatula. Bake for 15 minutes or until the crust is golden brown.
4. Spread the tomato sauce over the dough using the back of a spoon. Pour the cheese on top.
5. Bake 10 more minutes or until pizza is golden brown.
6. Sprinkle oregano on top and serve.

Low carb fresh asparagus salad
Extra recipe for meal replacement

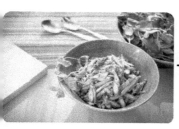

Time 10 + 10 m | easy

I love asparagus, especially when it comes from Peru, one of the world's leading asparagus producers. Today we are going to serve them raw, with all their nutrients, in a wonderful and fresh salad that will surprise everyone

Ingredients

20 ml chopped walnuts

3 oz. fresh green asparagus

$1/6$ lemons, zest and juice

$1/6$ flakes dash of chili spicy

$1/6$ tsp. Salt

10 ml avocado oil

⅓ tbsp. olive oil

20 ml grated parmesan cheese

Instructions

1. Preheat the oven to 350º F / 175º C. Roast the chopped walnuts until lightly browned, about 10 minutes

2. While the walnuts are in the oven, cut the asparagus into very thin slices. You can angle the knife to make the task easier. Eliminate the lower part that is usually harder.

3. Put the lemon zest and juice in a bowl. Add the hot pepper flakes, salt, avocado oil, and olive oil

4. Add the grated Parmesan and mix well

5. Take the asparagus in strips to the container and add the toasted walnuts. Integrate the salad well in smooth movements, using a rubber spatula

6. Garnish the salad with mint leaves and serve immediately

Low carb meatloaf
Extra recipe for meal replacement

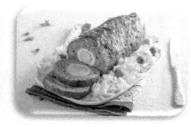

Time 20 + 40 m | medium difficulty

A dish that seems festive, attractive, tasty, and easy to prepare. For this I have been inspired by Colombian albodigón, although similar dishes can be found in several Latin American countries.

Ingredients

1/3 tbsp. room temperature butter, divided

1/6 lb ground beef (minced meat)

1/6 lb ground pork

2/5 tsp. Salt

1/6 tbsp. garlic powder

1/6 tbsp. onion powder

1/24 tsp. cumin seeds

1 / 10 tsp. Dried oregano

1 / 10 tsp. Cayenne pepper

2/3 oz red bell peppers, finely chopped

1/3 tbsp. chopped fresh parsley

1 chopped black olives

2/3 hard-boiled and peeled eggs

1/3 raw egg

At your service

1/3 oz chopped iceberg lettuce

1 pitted olives

fresh parsley for garnish

Instructions

1. Place a piece of waxed paper on the counter (approx. 13 "[33 cm]) long. Paint the paper with a quarter of the butter.

2. In a deep bowl, mix the beef, pork, salt, garlic powder, onion powder, cumin, oregano, cayenne pepper, red pepper, parsley, olive, a tablespoon of butter, and the raw eggs.

3. Mix with your hands, kneading until everything is mixed well. Spread this mixture on the waxed paper in a rectangle (approx. 11 "x 8" [28 x 20 cm]).

4. Place the eggs on the meat, and roll by centering the eggs on the roll and sealing the ends.

5. Wrap the meatloaf in the waxed paper and twist the ends of the paper to seal well. Place on a baking sheet.

6. Bake at 350ºF [175ºC] for 20 minutes

7. Remove from the oven, unwrap, discard the waxed paper and any juices that have accumulated on the tray (being careful not to break the meatloaf, or burn yourself!).

8. Brush the meatloaf with the remaining butter, increase the oven temperature to 200ºC [400ºF], and return the meatloaf to the oven for another 10 minutes

9. Remove from the oven and let it rest for five minutes. Serve surrounded by lettuce and garnished with olives and parsley.

Ketogenic Pizza
Extra recipe for meal replacement

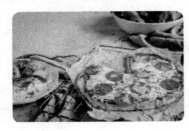

Time 5 + 25 m | easy

Let us introduce you: pizza, keto; keto, pizza ... This simple recipe is a great way to enjoy a pizza without the carbohydrates. It has everything important: pepperoni, cheese, and tomato sauce. Delicious!

Ingredients Base

2 eggs

¾ taza (3 oz.) mozzarella cheese, grated

Coverage

1 ½ tbsp. unsweetened tomato sauce

½ tsp. Dried oregano

2/3 cup grated provolone cheese or mozzarella cheese

¾ oz. pepperoni

olives (optional)

At your service

½ cup leafy greens

2 tbsp. olive oil

sea salt and ground black pepper

Instructions

1. Preheat the oven to 200 ° C (400 ° F)

2. Start by making the dough. Add the eggs to a medium bowl and add the grated cheese. Stir well to mix.

3. Use a spatula to spread the cheese and beaten eggs onto a cookie sheet lined with greaseproof paper. You can form two circles or just make a large rectangle-shaped pizza. Bake 15 minutes until the dough is golden brown. Remove from the oven and let it cool for a minute or two.

4. Raise the oven temperature to 450 ° F (225 ° C).

5. Spread the tomato paste on the base and sprinkle oregano on top. Add the cheese and top with the pepperoni and olives.

6. Bake for another 5-10 minutes or until the pizza is golden brown.

7. Serve with a fresh salad.

5
+
2
5
m
|
e
a
s

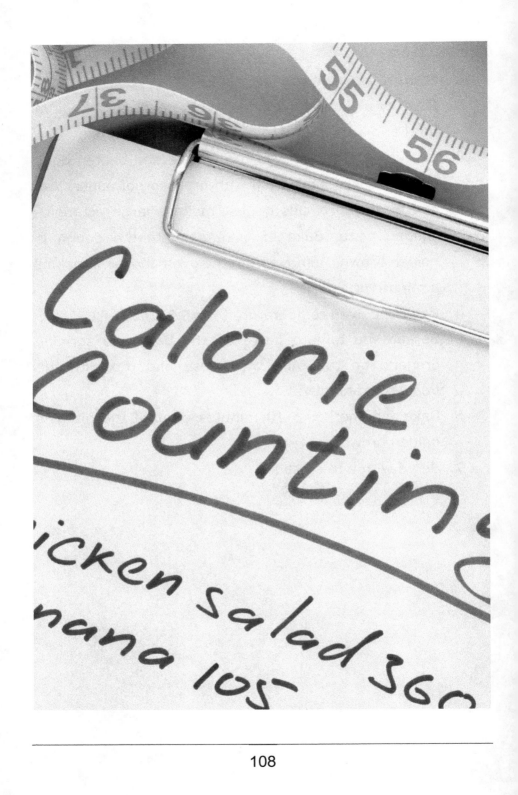

Calorie
Counting

icken salad 360
nana 105

Chapter 12:

Why We Do Not Recommend Counting Calories

First of all, it is impossible to know exactly how many calories you will get from a specific food, much less to know precisely what the body will do with those calories. It is much more important to choose foods that promote the release of hormones that reduce hunger, that help us stay full, and that makes it easier to achieve a healthy weight.

We should focus on authentic foods that contain good quality protein, healthy fats, and nutrient-rich fibrous carbohydrates, especially vegetables that grow on the surface.

If you're having a hard time losing weight, refrain from high-calorie, rewarding foods-it's easy to lose control, even if they're low in carbs. Some classic examples are cheese and nuts.

Instead of counting calories, make all calories count: eat low-carb, nutritious, and balanced foods.

I don't recommend counting calories. After fasting, I would try to eat as normally as possible. It would be like a normal dinner, but maybe with a slightly larger portion size.

Remember that protein consumption on a fasting day will be much lower than normal. On meal day, you can simply compensate by eating more, although most people eat at least 3-4 times more protein than they need for normal health.

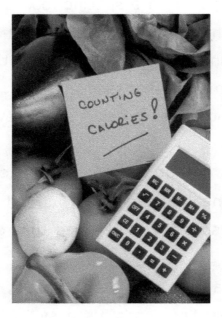

Chapter 11:

What Happens When You Don't Eat For 24 Hours? Myth vs. Reality

Myth 1: Your Metabolism Slows Down

This idea has its origin in studies with mice, but there are two problems:

A mouse has a short life (2-3 years). A fast of a day in a mouse would perhaps equal more than a week in a human.

Mice have very little fat and are more sensitive to caloric deficits. On the contrary, humans are mammals with more% fat.

Interestingly, in us, fasting causes a slight increase in metabolism, partly because of the release of norepinephrine and orexin. It is an evolutionary adaptation: motivation to go hunting.

Of course, a prolonged fast will slow the metabolism. It is logical, knowing that leptin takes several days to reduce enough the hypothalamus tendency to react, regulating downward energy expenditure.

As we saw in this book, what slows down the metabolism is precisely a prolonged period of a hypocaloric diet, just what they recommend.

Myth 2: Burn Muscle

When your body has consumed all the amino acids in the blood and stored glycogen, it starts using protein stores, your muscles, to convert them into glucose (via gluconeogenesis). You should avoid this process, but fortunately, it does not happen in the first 24 hours of fasting. A couple of examples:

A study concludes that intermittent fasting retains more muscle mass than a traditional hypocaloric approach (with similar fat loss).

Another study with intermittent fasting in obese adults found that it is effective for weight loss, even increasing muscle mass. This study also compared intermittent fasting with a high-fat approach (45% of total calories) against another moderate in fat (25% of total calories). The high fat achieved greater muscle gain and fat loss. Interesting.

One possible limitation of these studies is that they are performed in overweight people, and we know that fat protects the muscle.

What would happen in people with a lot of muscle and low fat?

According to this study in Muslim bodybuilders, fasting during the month of Ramadan does not result in loss of muscle mass. Women who trained strength with intermittent fasting (16/8) gained the same amount of muscle as those who did more meals, but they lost some more fat.

It may be due in part to the increase in growth hormone generated by fasting, the protective role of autophagy, and the reduction of myostatin, which inhibits muscle development.

Supplement companies invest a lot of money in promoting the need to ingest 20g of protein every 3 hours. Their dream would be for everyone to drink protein shakes on snacks. It is not necessary.

But more is not better; a prolonged fast is dangerous for the muscle. Your tolerance level will depend on the accumulated glycogen and physical activity performed, but in general, I do not recommend frequent fasting for more than 24-36 hours. Run away from detox diets for a week, for example.

Myth 3: Low Sugar

The body is designed to maintain the proper level of blood glucose. When you eat you produce insulin to store excess glucose. When you fast you produce glucagon to release stored glucose. Eating frequently to control blood glucose externally is not necessary. You can dedicate your time to more productive things.

Intermittent fasting helps restore sensitivity to a greater extent than classical calorie restriction in people with insulin resistance.

In another study, people with type II diabetes responded better to two large meals a day than six small ones. We also know that intermittent fasting is effective against metabolic problems.

Myth 4: You Will Not Give Up in Training

The impact of fasting on performance depends on many factors, such as the type of physical activity, the duration of fasting, and the level of adaptation. Still, there are many examples where this loss of performance does not materialize, once adopted.

Reviews of studies in Muslim athletes during Ramadan show inconsistent results. Resistance tests are most affected, but it is necessary to consider that during Ramadan the fluids are also restricted during the day, so it is difficult to know what effect is due to fasting and which is due to daily dehydration. In any case, the variations are small.

The truth is that fasting training (with low glycogen) favors adaptations that would not occur if you always train with full reserves.

And finally, a recent study in strength athletes demonstrates that an intermittent fasting strategy not only maintains muscle performance and gains, but is more effective in losing fat. The same happens in women; this study concludes.

Myth 5: You Will Be Hungry, Headaches, and Irritation

It is possible that all this happens the first time. Like everything, it is a matter of adaptation.

But there is much evidence against distributing food in many small intakes:

A study concluded that increasing the frequency of meals increases hunger; while another suggested that it can promote a higher caloric intake.

My experience: the most important thing to improve adherence (and therefore success) is to be satiated when you eat. If you eat 1,800 calories a day and divide it into 6 intakes, you have 300 calories left over. Result: constant hunger. Compressing the feeding window reduces appetite.

Regarding irritation, it is subjective, but some studies indicate that intermittent fasting improves mood and symptoms of depression and improves mental alertness. Personally, it would irritate me much more to have to prepare six meals a day and never be satiated. Intermittent fasting represents great mental and time release.

Myth 6: You Will Gain Weight

Simply absurd. Multiple studies show that intermittent fasting helps you lose fat better than classic hypocaloric diets. Recent reviews already recognize it as an effective strategy to lose weight.

The justification of some is that by skipping one meal you will accumulate hunger and you will eat twice as much at the next meal, but we know that does not happen.

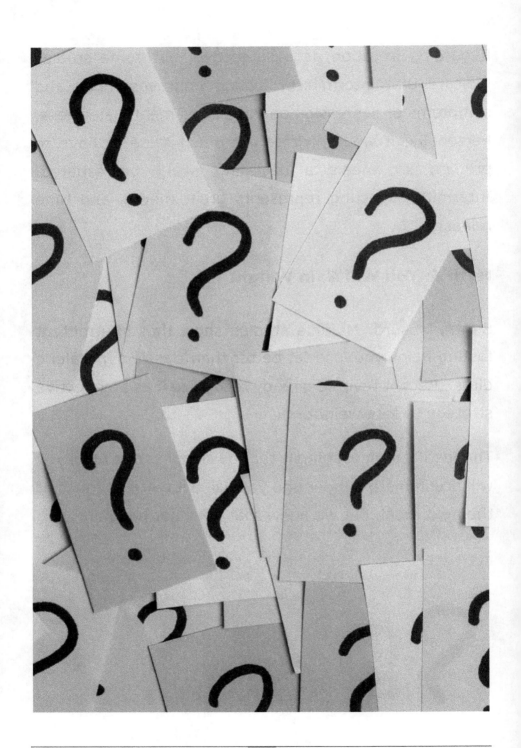

Chapter 13:

Frequently asked questions and answers about fasting

Who should NOT fast?

You should not fast in the following cases:

⇒ If you are underweight or have an eating disorder such as anorexia.

⇒ If you are pregnant: you need more nutrients for the baby.

⇒ If you are breastfeeding: you need more nutrients for the baby.

⇒ If you are under 18: you need more nutrients to grow.

And in the following situations, you can fast, but you may need medical supervision:

⇒ If you have type 1 or type 2 diabetes.

⇒ If you take medications that have been prescribed for you.

⇒ If you have gout or high uric acid.

⇒ If you have serious medical conditions such as liver disease, kidney disease, or heart disease.

Won't fasting put me in a state of starvation?

No. This is the most common myth about intermittent fasting, and it's generally not true.

Some studies indicate that intermittent fasting may even increase basal metabolic rate (at least initially) and may improve overall body composition.

Can I exercise while fasting?

⇒ Yes, while fasting you can continue to do all of your usual activities, including exercise.

⇒ You do not need to have eaten recently to provide the energy you need for exercise.

⇒ Instead, your body can burn stored energy (such as body fat) for energy.

⇒ However, for long-duration aerobic exercise, eating before exercise may increase performance.

⇒ Keep in mind that it is important to drink fluids and replenish sodium (salt) when you exercise on an empty stomach.

What are the possible side effects?

Several uncomfortable side effects can occur.

What to do if you are in pain:

⇒ Hunger is the most common side effect of intermittent fasting. It can be less of a problem if you're already on a keto diet or a low-carb, high-fat diet.
⇒ Constipation is a common occurrence. Let's just say that if the less gets into your body, the less will get out. Keep in mind that this is a natural response to eating less. There is no need to worry and no treatment is needed except if there is significant bloating or abdominal discomfort. If needed, regular laxatives or magnesium supplements can be taken to help.
⇒ Headaches are common and usually disappear after the first few fasts.
Often consuming a little more salt will help mitigate them.

⇒ Mineral water can help in case the stomach is rumbling.

⇒ Other possible side effects include dizziness, heartburn, and muscle cramps.

Since most of these side effects are manageable, however, if you feel sick, dizzy, feel completely weak, or have other serious symptoms, then you should stop the fast. Just remember to come out of the fast calmly and slowly, prioritizing liquids and salt (bone broth is a great way to start). And, of course, if symptoms persist, you should visit your doctor immediately. Fortunately, serious side effects occur very rarely, and even less so if you stay well hydrated and supplement with electrolytes.

Why does blood sugar rise during fasting?

Although this doesn't happen to everyone, blood sugar can rise, and this is due to hormonal changes that occur during fasting. The body produces sugar to provide energy to the system. This is a variation of the sunrise phenomenon and is generally nothing to worry about as long as blood sugar levels do not remain high for the rest of the day.

What do I do if I'm hungry?

The most important thing is to know that hunger passes quickly. Many people worry that the hunger they feel during intermittent fasting will increase to unbearable levels, but that's not what happens.

If you ignore it and have a cup of tea or coffee, it will often pass, even better if you have a sugar-free lemonade.

During long fasts, it is common for hunger to intensify on the second day. Then it gradually diminishes, and many people experience a complete lack of appetite on the third or fourth day.

The body is now feeding on fat. The body is "eating" its fat at breakfast, lunch, and dinner, so it is not hungry.
Won't fasting cause me to burn muscle?
This depends on each person and the length of the fast. During fasting, the body first breaks down glycogen into glucose to use as energy. Then it increases the breakdown of fat to provide energy. Excess amino acids (the building blocks of protein) are also used for energy, but the body does not burn its muscle unless it has to.

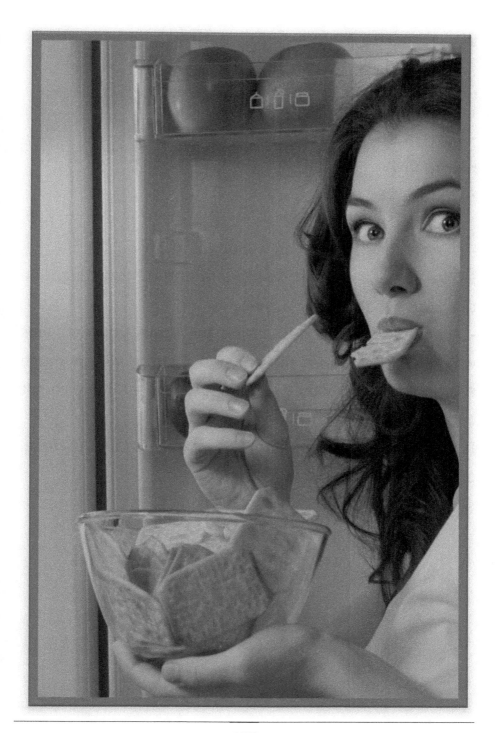

What are the main tips for fasting?

Here are the top seven tips, summarized:

- Drink water
- Keep busy
- Drink coffee or tea

- Don't think about being hungry
- Give yourself a month to see if intermittent fasting (like the 16:8 type) is right for you
- Follow a low-carb diet during the times you eat. This way you will be less hungry and fasting will be much easier. And your body will no longer feel the need to eat carbs and sugars
It will also increase the effect of weight loss and reversal of type 2 diabetes, etc.

Don't binge after fasting

How to get out of a fast?

Slowly. The longer the fast, the more carefully it needs to be ended.

After fast, many people make the mistake of eating a big meal this will produce stomachache. Fasting will teach you to eat more gradually and normally without making big binges.

Isn't it important to eat breakfast every day?
Not necessarily. This is a misconception based on speculation and statistics, but it doesn't hold up when put to the test.

Skipping breakfast gives your body more time to burn fat and use it as energy. Because you're less hungry in the morning, it's often easier to skip it and break the fast later in the day.

Can women fast?

Yes, with some exceptions. Those who should not fast are women who are underweight, pregnant or breastfeeding.

Beyond that, women who are trying to conceive (and perhaps even more specifically for athletic women with a low body fat percentage) should be aware that intermittent fasting may increase the risk of irregular periods and reduce the chance of conceiving.

Aside from these reasons, there is no particular reason why women should not fast.

Isn't fasting the same as cutting calories?

Not necessarily. Fasting shortens the time you eat and primarily answers the question of "when to eat?"

Cutting calories answers the question "what and how much to eat?" These are different topics and should not be confused with each other.

There may be a reduction in calories in fasting, but its benefits go beyond that.

Will I lose weight with intermittent fasting?

Most likely, yes.

If you have weight to lose, you will likely lose weight if you don't eat.

In theory, it is possible that after fasting you will eat more and gain the weight you lost. However, studies show that people

who fast tend to eat a lot less and be more conscientious in what they eat.

CPSIA information can be obtained
at www.ICGtesting.com
Printed in the USA
LVHW031337130721
692557LV00010B/936

9 781803 120928